Retained Neonatal Reflexes

a revolutionary approach to treating children
with learning difficulties and behavioural problems

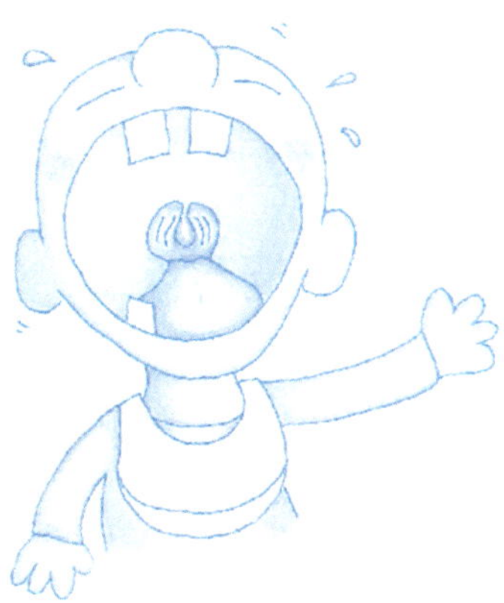

Dr. Susan Walker
Doctor of Chiropractic

Contents

Welcome

At this clinic we can ensure your healthcare is tailored to your body's individual requirements.

Working with people in all phases of life, from newborns to the elderly, we have found Chiropractic care to be an extremely safe and effective way to maintain your family's health.

We focus on establishing ideal nervous system function to improve learning, behaviour, muscle tone and body control. Intrigued by the complexities of the human body, Professional Applied Kinesiology (PAK) Chiropractors are able to assess and then treat a multitude of contributing causes of a health concern.

Your practitioner will use their knowledge of the

- muscular system to make moving easier by strengthening the muscles which stabilise your joints and enhance your co-ordination so you can use your body more efficiently
- nervous system so your brain communicates with your body, and your body can give feedback to your brain unimpeded
- craniosacral system to assist your cerebrospinal fluid to supply nourishment to your nervous system as it circulates around your brain and down your spinal cord
- acupuncture system to ensure free and balanced energetic flow around your body
- biochemical processes, energy production, and hormones to enable your body to function at its best.

What is Chiropractic?

Chiropractic is based on the scientific fact that your body is a self-regulating, self-healing organism. All bodily functions are controlled by the brain, spinal cord and nerves throughout the body.

Specialised tissues in the nervous system release chemical messengers in the form of neurotransmitters and hormones. These chemicals are a means of communication to and from the brain and body so are essential for maintaining perfect balance between the body's organ systems.

The moving bones of the spine and skull protect the vulnerable communication pathways of the brain, spinal cord and nerves. The movement is also essential for the transportation of these chemical messengers. If the nervous system is impaired it can cause malfunction of the tissues and organs throughout the body. For this reason, most often, when thinking about Chiropractic, we think of adjustments to the spine but it really does incorporate a lot more.

The delicate tissues of your brain are protected by the 28 bones that make up your skull:
- ▶ 8 that form the cranial vault to house the brain
- ▶ 14 that make up the face
- ▶ and 6 in your ears that allow you to hear.

Since the majority of your nervous system begins above the spine, in your brain, our Chiropractors assess and perform corrections for cranial faults when skull movement or position is impaired. This is commonly needed after long labours or traumatic births, or simply bumps to the head. However it also may be required after dental work, teeth grinding or to assist in the correction of long-standing postural problems.

There are also 33 vertebrae that make up the spinal column in a child, which fuse to 24 by adulthood. Your spinal cord runs through the centre of these bones, which allows your body to have flexible movement while your most precious structures are being safely protected within.

Optimum alignment of your bones is essential to
stream your brain's messages to your body and your
body's feedback to your brain.

Optimal alignment of your skull and spinal bones
enhances concentration, vitality, strength and agility
... and that's why you feel so terrific after your
Chiropractic adjustments!

What is Professional Applied Kinesiology (PAK)?

Chiropractic is the science of locating offending spinal
structures, the art of reducing their impact on the
nervous system and a philosophy of natural health care
based on your inborn potential to be healthy.
PAK is a diagnostic system whereby muscle patterns
are tested and interpreted by a skilled practitioner to
assist in determining what type of care a patient needs.

PAK provides immediate feedback to enable the
correct application of treatment for you. This way your
practitioner can judge from your muscle responses if
a certain correction will be therapeutic for you. This
method works by detecting subtle changes in the
function of your nervous system when it is challenged,
or stressed, by different stimuli.

Professional Applied Kinesiology (PAK) is a trademarked
term used around the world reserved for use only
by primary healthcare professionals who have been
formally trained in the skills of Applied Kinesiology.

For more information about Professional Applied Kinesiology visit:
www.icaka.org.au

Retained Neonatal Reflexes™

The Retained Neonatal Reflexes technique is a revolutionary approach to helping children and adults with learning difficulties and behavioural problems.

Founded in Australia by Chiropractor Dr. Keith Keen in the early 1990s, the past two decades have seen the RNR technique develop to incorporate corrections for more than a dozen retained neonatal reflexes. These corrections are aimed to assist in the integration and to normalise the aberrant display of retained primitive and neonatal reflexes.

What is a Retained Neonatal Reflex?

In the womb and in early life, when the decision making process has not fully developed, your brainstem has several reflexes called 'primitive' reflexes. After birth these reflexes can be referred to as 'neonatal' reflexes. They help you grow properly and safely. For example, they help you in the birthing process, with breast feeding and with gripping onto things.

As you mature these reflexes are no longer needed. So they take a 'back seat' and the higher brain takes control. This is a normal and essential stage of your development. However, due to birth trauma or developmental restrictions, these reflexes might remain dominant. This means that your nervous system will automatically react inappropriately and undesirably in certain situations. This can adversely affect your development, learning and behaviour. This is a *Retained Neonatal Reflex*.

Using specific techniques developed by Australian Chiropractors and now taught all over the world, we can assist in the integration of these reflexes that could be holding you or your bright children back.

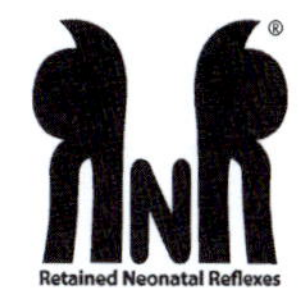

To find a qualified RNR practitioner near you visit:
www.retainedneonatalreflexes.com.au

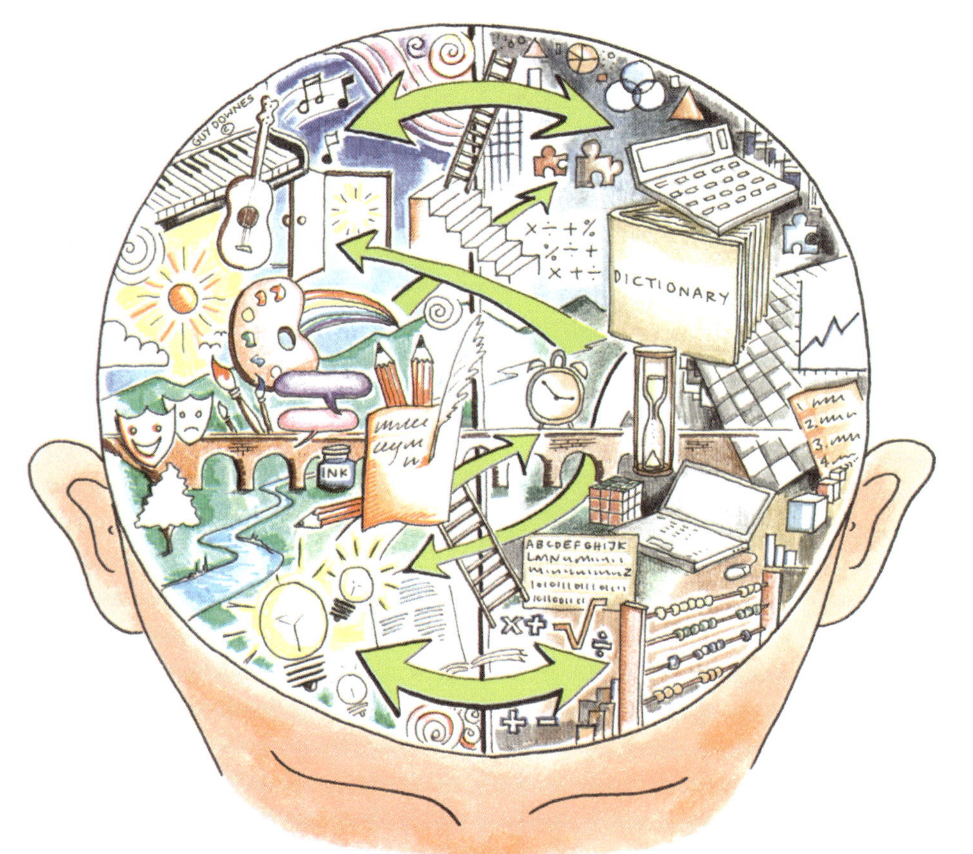

GUY DOWNES ©
DICTIONARY
INK
x ÷ + %
% ÷ +
x ÷
ABCDEFGHIJK
LMN   Z
X +   √   ÷
+ −

Hemispheres

Your brain is a collective of around 100 billion nerves assembled in a brilliantly organised design. These nerves are compartmentalized into several sections or segments; the largest of which is formed by a fissure that divides the upper brain into two distinct halves. These two half brains are called the cerebral hemispheres, one on the left and one on the right, and they communicate via a thick band of connecting nerves between them.

The left and right hemispheres have very different responsibilities. Generally, one hemisphere will give signals to, and receive information from, the opposite side of the body. For example, when your right arm moves, the movement is controlled by your left hemisphere, and when your right arm is being touched, it is the left side of your brain that interprets the sensation.

The left brain is known for being the most logical hemisphere engaging for tasks such as language, mathematics and knowledge, whereas your right brain is considered the more creative hemisphere used for imagination, music and philosophy.

As practitioners working with the nervous system and overall function of the body, we recognise the importance of minimizing dominance in the function of one particular hemisphere and we have methods of assisting the balance of function.

Hemispheric dysfunction may lead to any of the following symptoms:

o Handedness - a clear preference for one hand over the other
o Sidedness - one ear, eye or side of the body dominates the other
o One sided weakness resulting in poor coordination (dyspraxia)
o Poor coordination between both sides of the body affecting sport, dance, play, etc.
o Difficulty processing school tasks such as adding numbers
o Reluctance to hum tunes
o Lack of creative ability

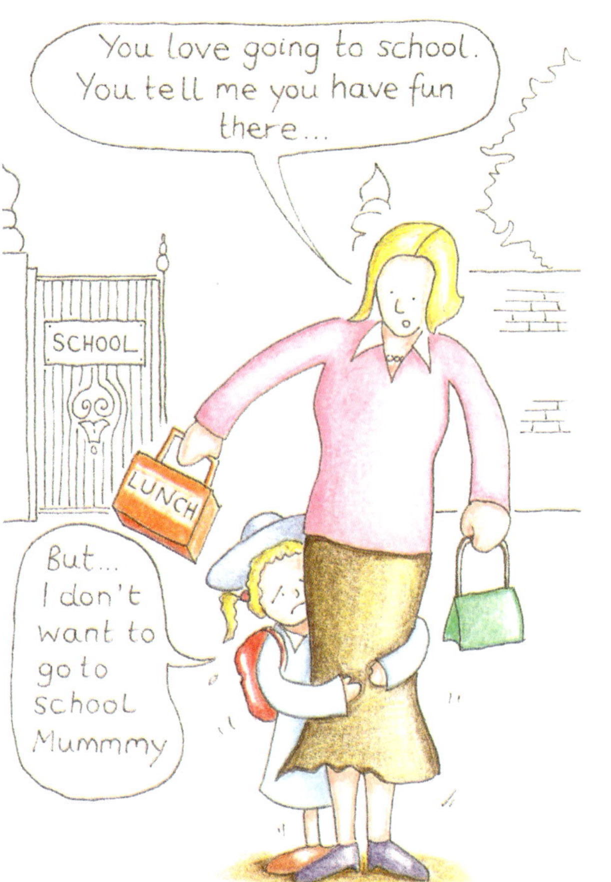

You love going to school. You tell me you have fun there...
SCHOOL
LUNCH
But... I don't want to go to school Mummmy

Fear Paralysis Reflex (FPR)

Inside each of us we have an impressive communication network that controls our body without us needing to think about it. There are more nerves in this network than there are stars in our universe. It is totally automatic and works all the time whether we are sleeping or awake. This special part of our wiring is called the Autonomic Nervous System or ANS for short.

There are two main parts of the ANS; one for emergencies that need us to 'fight' or 'take flight', the other for when we 'rest' and 'digest' which alows us build up and save energy for the next emergency. The two parts need to be in balance and when the FPR is retained the balance shifts excessively towards 'rest and digest'.

When still in the womb, the Fear Paralysis Reflex temporarily causes a cessation of the baby's movement if the mother is ever under threat. If this reflex is retained, you could feel 'butterflies in your belly' if placed in an uncomfortable situation. Excessive worry or anxiety are terms used to describe this feeling and the ensuing behaviour. A retained FPR can be responsible for the 'deer in headlights' effect whe stunned, and can make us move slower and more cautiously when we're uncertain of our surroundings.

Retained Fear Paralysis Reflex may lead to any of the following symptoms:

- Anxiety seemingly unrelated to reality
- Low tolerance to stress
- Temper tantrums
- Hypersensitivity to touch, sound or changes in visual field
- Dislike of change or surprise
- Poor adaptability
- Fatigue
- Breath holding
- Fear of social embarrassment
- Insecurity / lack of trust in oneself
- Overly clingy or may be unable to accept or demonstrate affection easily
- Compulsive traits / Obsessive Compulsive Disorder
- Negativity or defeatist attitude
- Won't try new activities, especially where comparison or excellence is expected
- Immediate motor paralysis under stress – can't think and move at the same time

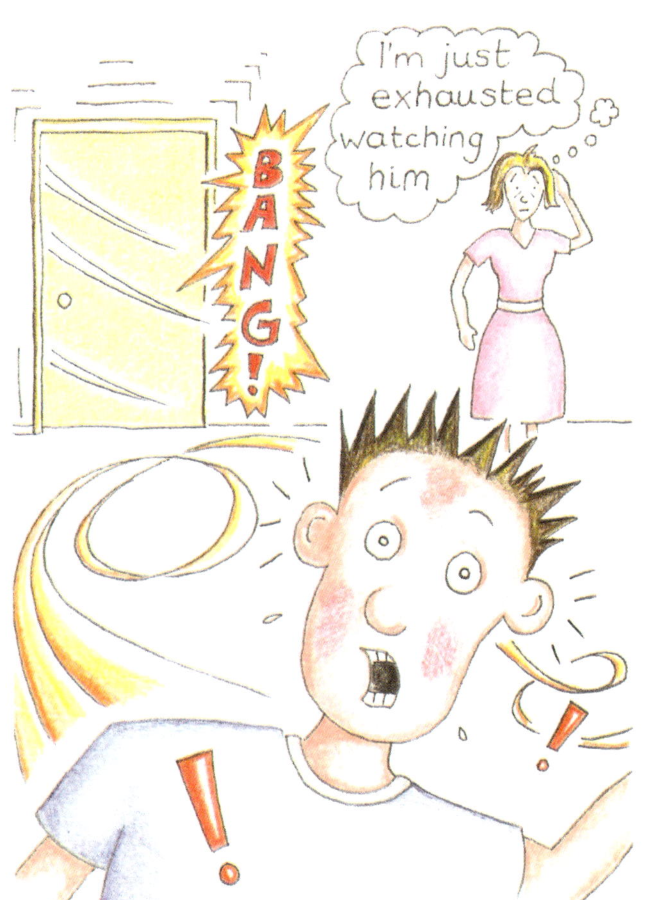
I'm just exhausted watching him
BANG!

Moro Reflex

A newborn baby's higher centres have not yet developed enough to make a rational decision about whether a circumstance is threatening or not. It is protected by an involuntary 'one reflex for all occasions', that is, one set of physical and hormonal events which cover for most eventualities.

The reflex is set off by excessive information in any of the baby's senses – for example, a loud noise, bright light, sudden rough touch, sudden stimulation of the balance mechanism such as dropping or tilting. It is the earliest form of the adrenal 'fight' or 'take flight' response. The adrenal glands are capable of giving your body the extreme energy rush you experience when you get a sudden surprise. This response prepares the body for fighting or running and if not integrated can lead to hyperactivity. As the adrenal glands are a large part of our immune system, constantly being 'turned on' can lead to adrenal fatigue and therefore asthma, allergies, and chronic illness.

Retained Moro Reflex may lead to:
o Hyperactivity
o Hypersensitivity to sudden noise, light or movement
o Difficulty with new or stimulating experiences
o Impulsive behaviour
o Distractibility – having to pay attention to everything
o Anxiety, particularly anticipation anxiety
o Emotional and social immaturity
o Sensitivity to foods or food additives
o Inappropriate behaviour
o Adrenal fatigue, leading to allergy, asthma or chronic illness

With a retained Moro Reflex, a child may never have fully experienced the discovery phase of development, otherwise known as *the terrible twos*. As the Moro integrates after treatment, the child (or teenager or adult) has the opportunity to pass through this important developmental phase. *Terrible twos* may not appear appropriate in later years, but it is important that this phase of development runs its course. Emotional ups and downs are common for a short period as the nervous system and hormonal system readjust, but then the benefits of correction shine through.

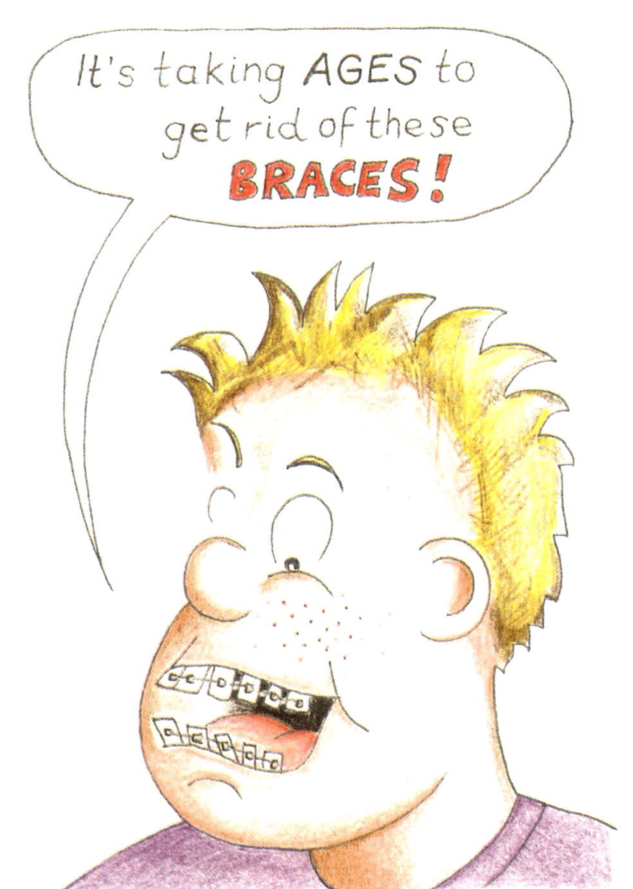

It's taking AGES to get rid of these BRACES!

Juvenile Suck Reflex

A newborn baby projects its tongue forward to suck a nipple. In the adult swallow reflex, the tongue moves backwards to push food down the throat.

If a Juvenile Suck Reflex is not adequately integrated, the tongue projects forwards before moving backward in the adult swallow. This tongue thrust continually pushes the front teeth forwards. This causes a narrow mouth arch and protruding upper teeth, one of the common problems requiring orthodontics.

Braces or a dental retainer may be required for longer periods when a Juvenile Suck Reflex is retained.

Retained Juvenile Suck Reflex may lead to:
- Speech and articulation problems
- Difficulty swallowing and chewing
- Difficulty speaking or chewing and doing manual tasks at the same time
- Involuntary tongue or mouth movements when writing or drawing
- Overbite of the upper jaw, requiring dental intervention

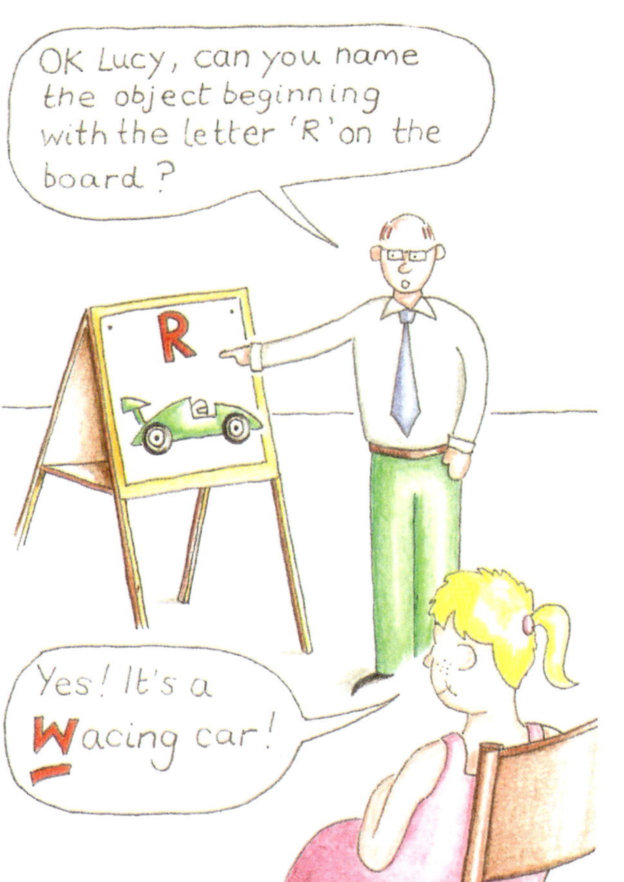

OK Lucy, can you name the object beginning with the letter 'R' on the board?
Yes! It's a Wacing car!

Rooting Reflex

Light touch of the cheek near the edge of the mouth will cause a baby to turn its head toward that side, open its mouth and extend the tongue in preparation for suckling. This reflex is named the Rooting Reflex.

If retained, there may be hypersensitivity around the lips and mouth. The tongue may remain too far forward, resulting in speech problems, dribbling, or difficulty swallowing and chewing. This may be seen with fussy eaters or thumb suckers.

This correction may promote normalization of hormonal functions in children and adults. Many cases with abnormal thyroid or adrenal tests have demonstrated improvements, and laboratory tests have moved to normal ranges after this correction. Most importantly, symptoms related to hormonal imbalance have cleared.

Retained Rooting Reflex may lead to:

- Dribbling
- Speech problems
- Hypersensitivity around lips and mouth
- Tongue sitting too far forward in the mouth
- Difficulty speaking or chewing and doing manual tasks at the same time
- Hormonal imbalances

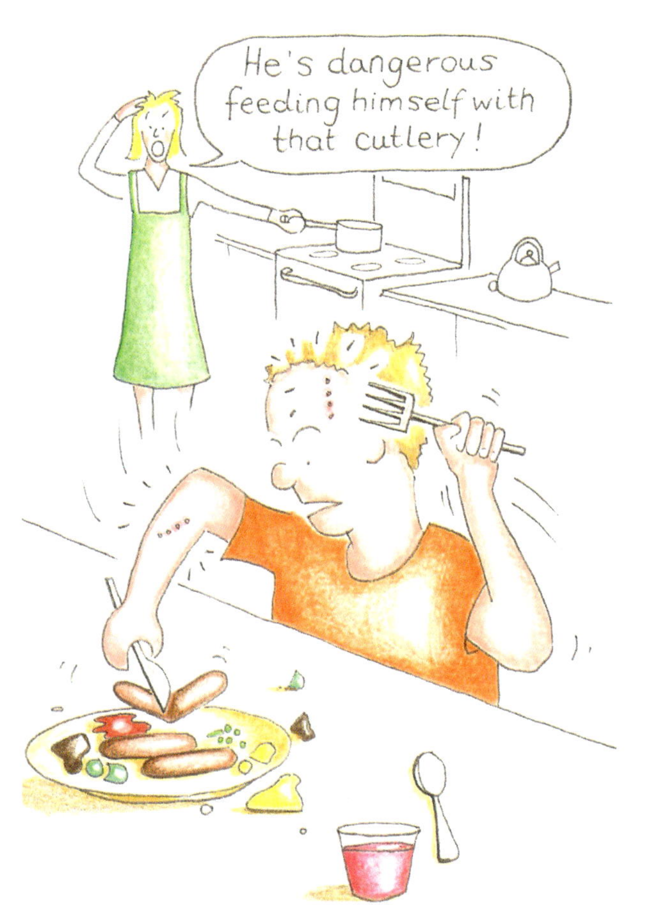

He's dangerous feeding himself with that cutlery!

Palmomental & Plantomental Reflex (PMR)

There is a link between the mouth and hands in the early months of life called the Babkin Response, seen as kneading movements of the hand associated with suckling. If this association remains, the patient may have a retained PMR. This is a two-way response; hand movement may affect speech and likewise movements of the mouth may affect the use of the hands. This relationship also creates contraction of muscles at the mouth when a portion of the hand is stimulated.

Due to the relationship between retention of this reflex and increased tension in the flexor muscles of the body, Carpal Tunnel Syndrome and tension in the calf muscles can resolve after the correction related to the retained PMR.

Retained PMR may lead to:

- A child's jaw opening and closing when using scissors
- Children biting others
- Difficulty learning to use cutlery
- Tight pencil grip
- Tension in facial muscles affecting facial expressions, which can influence stuttering
- Clenching the jaw whilst gripping a steering wheel

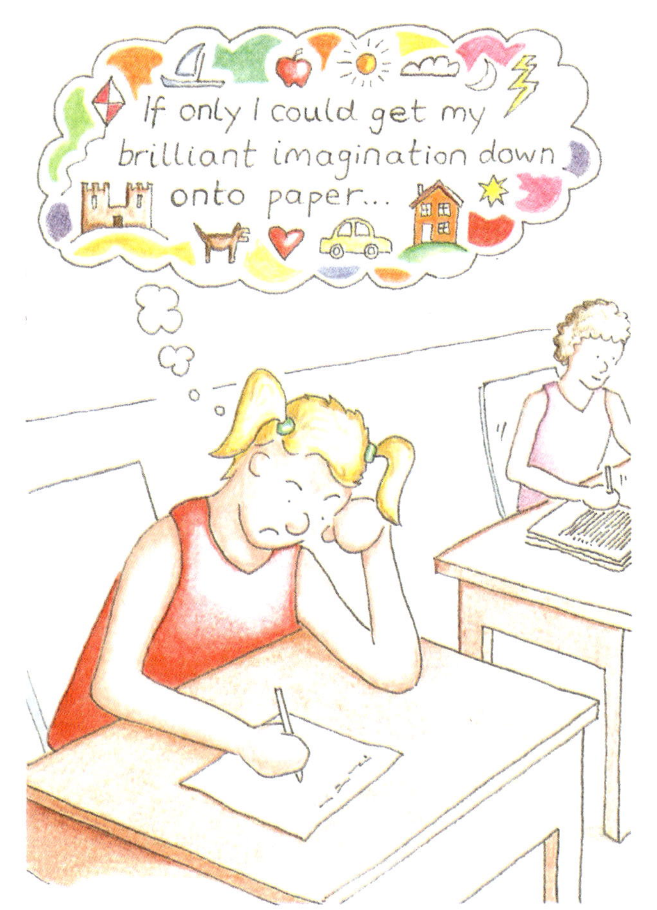

If only I could get my brilliant imagination down onto paper...

Palmar Reflex

Normal newborn babies have an active Palmar or Grasp Reflex. When the palm of the hand is touched, the three or four small fingers flex toward the palm to grasp. This grasp reflex must integrate to allow for the normal transition to the pincer grip, which then matures further allowing each finger to individually contact the thumb.

If retained, children often have poor handwriting and, more importantly, a poor ability to process their ideas and then write them down. That is, copying words is easy but the task of spelling words is more difficult and messy.

Independent movement of the fingers will tend to weaken other muscles of the body. Thus the child may slump during tasks like playing piano or making models. In an adult, he or she may complain that 'my back hurts when I sit in front of my computer', as typing requires independent finger movement.

Palmar Reflex retention may lead to:
- Poor fine motor skills and awkward use of hands
- Inappropriate pencil grip and poor handwriting
- Poor posture when playing piano or working with the hands
- Difficulty processing ideas on to paper or computer
- Poor posture and/or back pain when working at a desk or computer.
- Difficulty spelling or writing

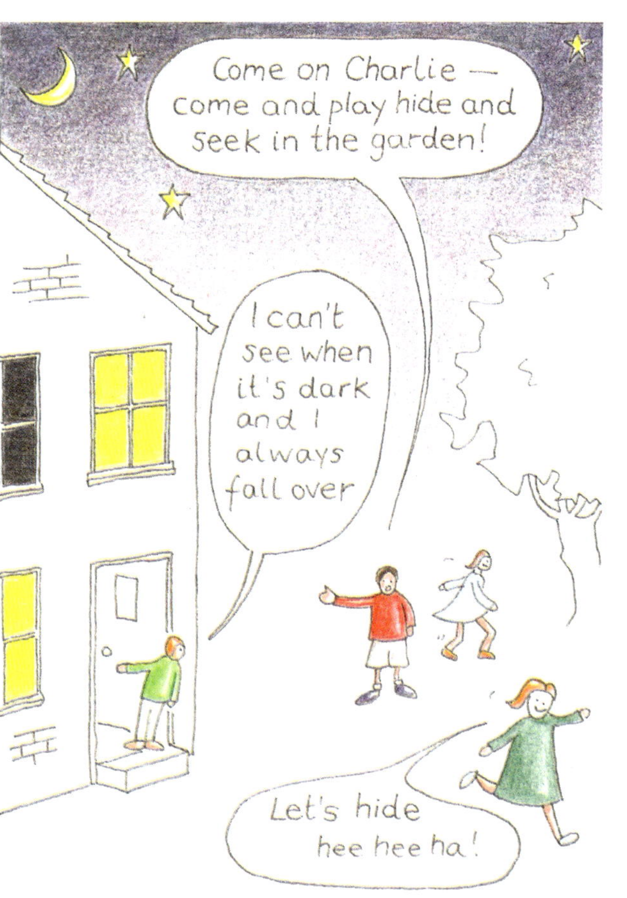

Come on Charlie — come and play hide and seek in the garden!
I can't see when it's dark and I always fall over
Let's hide hee hee ha!

Plantar Reflex

The Plantar Reflex is similar to the Palmar Reflex in that stroking or pressing on the underside of the foot causes the foot to flex and the toes to curl, as if to grasp whatever touched the foot.

We gather a great deal of information required for balance from our feet. We rely on independent movement of our toes to keep us steady and balanced. By improving the feedback to the intrinsic muscles of the feet, the muscles supporting the ankles, knees, hips and lower back don't have to overwork to keep balanced.

This reflex is commonly regained from long term disuse after injury and from the use of inappropriate footwear.

Plantar Reflex retention may lead to:

o Difficulty learning to walk
o Poor balance
o Toes curling under when putting on shoes causing difficulty getting the foot into shoes.
o Problems with sports requiring balance and co-ordination while running
o Lower back pain while walking and/or standing
o Recurring ankle twisting or shin soreness
o Difficulty walking in the dark (feet alone cannot properly maintain balance – vision is required to assist and, of course, vision cannot assist balance in the dark)

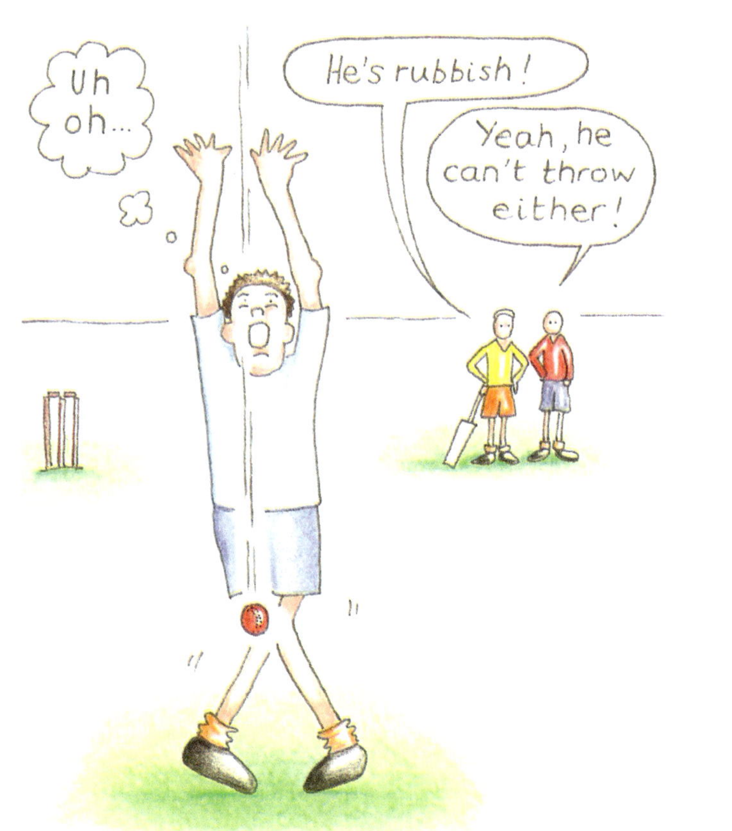

Uh oh...
He's rubbish!
Yeah, he can't throw either!

Asymmetrical Tonic Neck Reflex (ATNR)

If a newborn's head is turned to one side, the arm and leg on the side to which the head is turned straighten, while the opposite arm and leg pull in. It should be fully present at birth and appears to assist the baby's active participation in the birthing process. When a newborn displays the ATNR their hand will move in conjunction with his or her head. This connection between touch, sight and vision helps to establish distance perception and hand-eye co-ordination.

If the ATNR is retained, the hand and eye want to move together, making it difficult to look up at a blackboard, or up at a computer, while writing. When walking, turning the head results in the straightening of the arm and leg on the same side, which may upset balance and normal walking. With a retained ATNR, looking at the hand tends to compromise the strength of other muscle groups, which can affect a child's ability to catch a ball or participate in other sporting activities. In the early months, the ATNR locks baby's vision on to anything which catches his or her attention. If inappropriately retained, the child (or adult) can be easily distracted by anything that attracts their gaze.

ATNR retention may lead to:

o Hand-eye co-ordination difficulty (needed for catching and throwing balls)
o Judgment of distance may be affected
o Poor handwriting or awkward pencil grip
o Balance may be disturbed
o Difficulty copying from a blackboard
o Inability to cross the vertical midline (for example, a right-handed child may find it difficult to write on the left side of the page)
o Discrepancy between spoken and written performance
o Disturbance of the development of visual tracking, so they may miss parts of a line when reading (leading to poor comprehension)
o Bilateral integration (integrated use of the two sides of the body) may be poor. This can affect sporting abilities
o Establishment of a dominant hand, eye or ear may be difficult
o In adults there can be chronic shoulder and/or neck problems

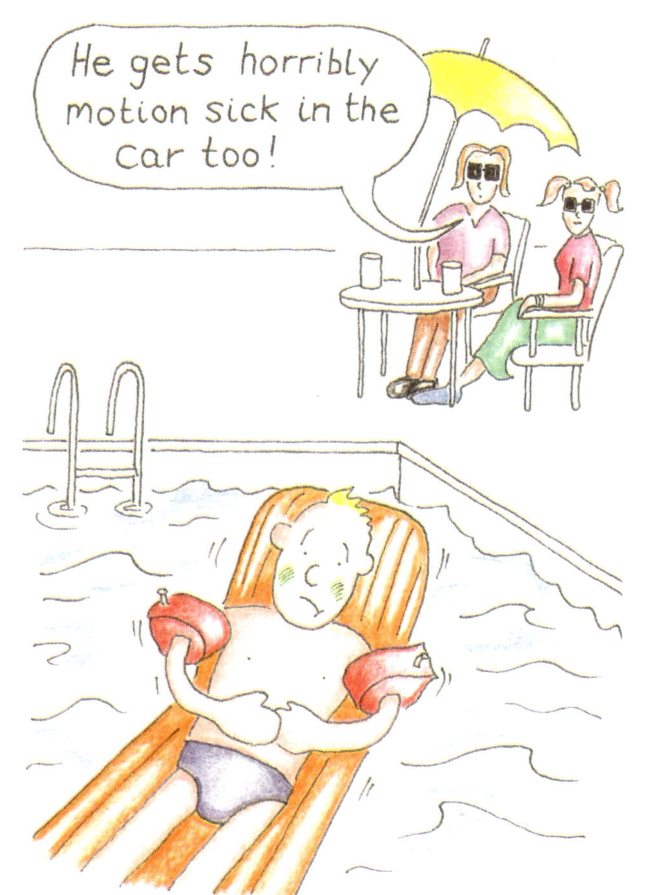

He gets horribly motion sick in the car too!

Tonic Labyrinthine Reflex (TLR)

TLR involves the vestibular system (the system provides a sense of balance and works out your position in space) and how it interacts with other senses. This allows your body to keep centred while you move.

A child who still has a retained TLR when starting to walk cannot acquire true standing and walking security and may experience difficulty in judging space, distance, depth and speed.

Retained Tonic Labyrinthine Reflex can be associated with:

- A 'floppy' child
- Poor balance
- Motion sickness
- Orientation and spatial difficulties
- Visual problems
- Difficulty judging space, distance, depth and speed

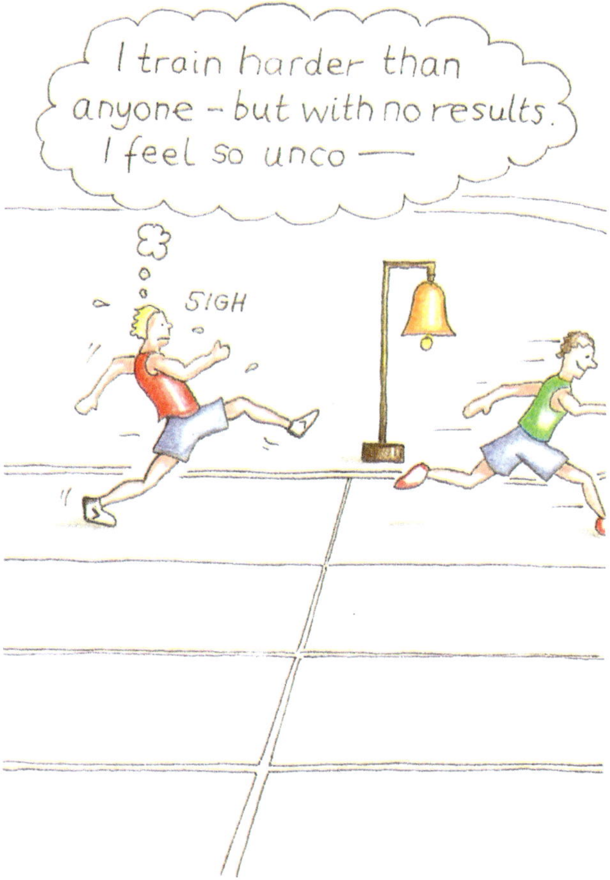

I train harder than anyone – but with no results. I feel so unco ——
SIGH

Sagittal Labyrinthine Reflex (SLR)

There are two main benefits related to the SLR correction. One helps concentration and posture when working over a desk. Another helps the body to co-ordinate movement, allowing it to move more efficiently.

Retained SLR makes concentrating difficult and very uncomfortable when working at a desk as the head hangs forward whilst sitting. Children are more likely to slump when sitting at a desk or a table, sit on their legs or generally twist and turn, resulting in what appears to be inattentiveness and possibly hyperactivity. They also tend to be quite slow at copying tasks.

It can also affect the integration of movement of the upper and lower limbs simultaneously, as in swimming or walking. These children are often diagnosed with dyspraxia (poor gross co-ordination) and can be seen by others as being clumsy. It is rare to see a patient fail to beat their personal best sporting performance after this correction has been performed.

Retained Sagittal Labyrinthine Reflex can be associated with:

o Poor concentration
o Fatigue while reading or when working or studying at a desk
o Bad posture when working over a desk
o Difficulty co-ordinating movement between arms and legs
o Sports performance below capability
o Difficulty kicking legs while simultaneously stroking arms when swimming

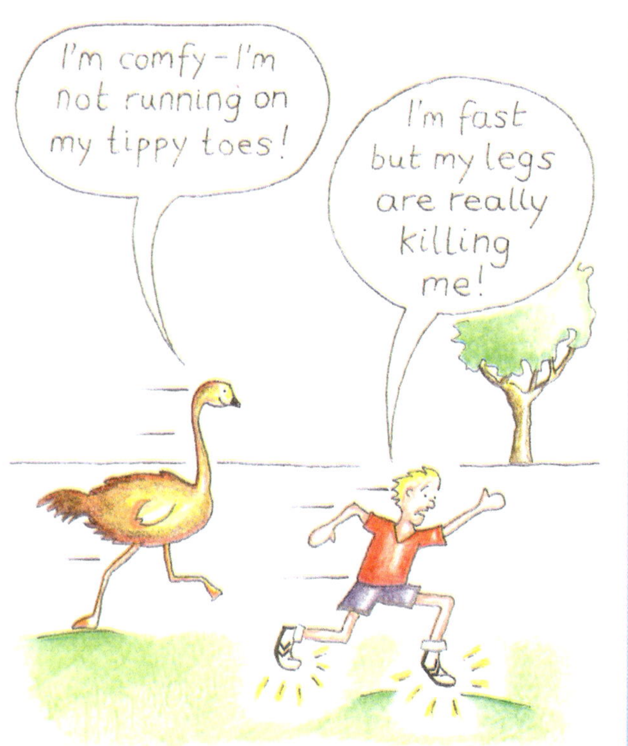

I'm comfy – I'm not running on my tippy toes!
I'm fast but my legs are really killing me!

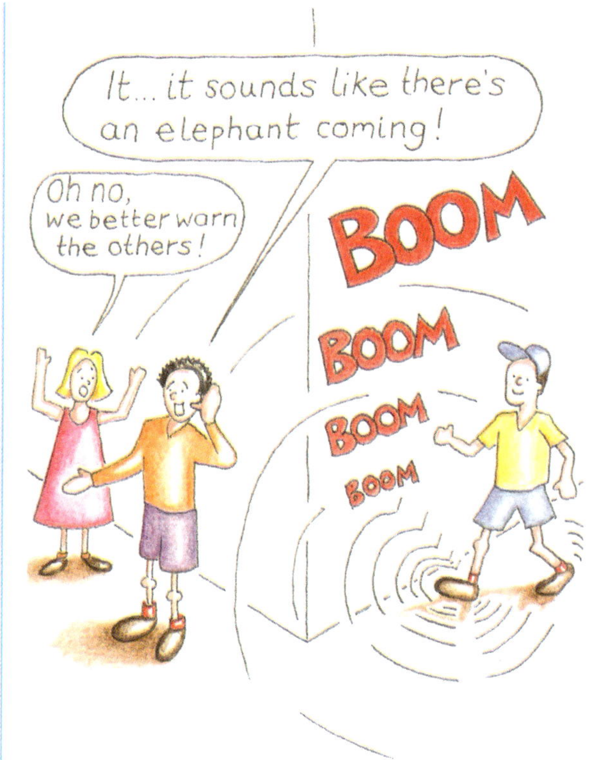

It... it sounds like there's an elephant coming!
Oh no, we better warn the others!
BOOM
BOOM
BOOM
BOOM

Stepping & Heel Reflexes

Our bodies alter our postural muscles depending if we are standing with our weight over our toes or our heels. These two reflexes help to remove tension from the muscles of the lower leg to allow for increased ankle movement, and establish ideal posture integrated with our vision.

A reasonable amount of the information we take in from our environment is through vision, so where we hold our head (tipping too far forward or back) has a tremendous influence on our posture. These two reflexes are aimed at balancing the connection between the input from our eyes and the feedback from our feet. Interestingly, many people retain both the Stepping and Heel reflexes.

Stepping Reflex retention may lead to:
o Toe walking – 'running like an ostrich'
o Tight calf muscles
o Poor balance and muscle control
o Feet and ankle problems with pain and dysfunction
o Recurring hamstring injuries and mid-low back strains
o Visual problems due to an altered perception of the horizon – head tilts forward and eyes look upward

Heel Reflex retention may lead to:
o Heavy heel walking – 'walking like an elephant'
o Heel pain, Achilles tendonitis, Shin splints
o Poor core stability
o Balance problems
o Visual problems due to an altered perception of the horizon – head tilts back and eyes look down

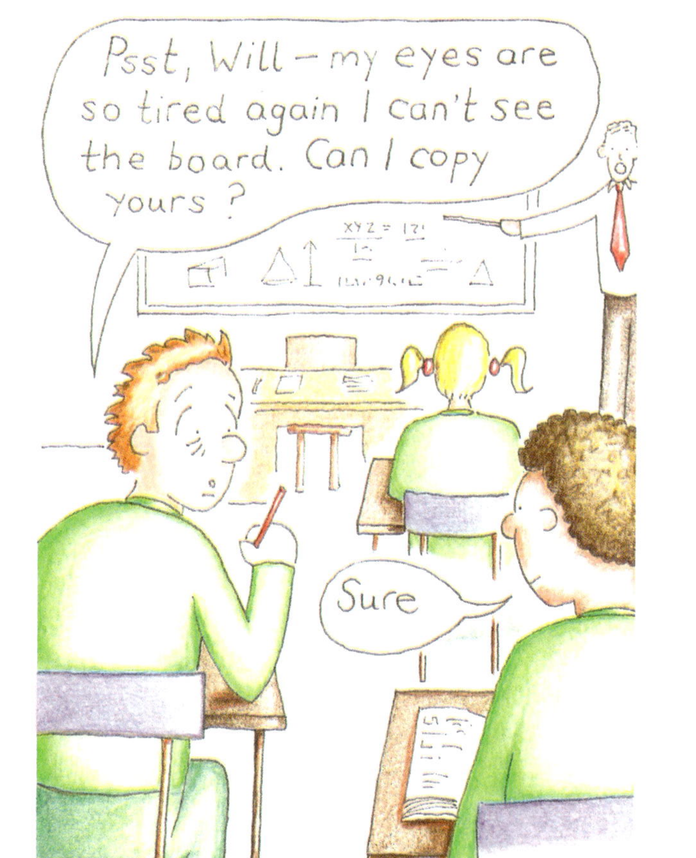

Psst, Will — my eyes are so tired again I can't see the board. Can I copy yours?
Sure

Symmetrical Tonic Neck Reflex (STNR)

The STNR is most evident just prior to crawling as the baby rocks forward and backward when on all fours.

When a baby is lying on his or her belly with straight legs and bent elbows, they flex their neck forward and their eyes focus on the floor. The baby can then straighten their arms, which reflexively tilts the head back and they focus their vision to the distance. At the same time their knees bend and they crouch.

This phase of development is important for refining near-far accommodation of the eyes, and therefore its correction can assist those whose eyes fatigue when copying things down off the blackboard or when driving (glancing from the road to the speedometer).

While it is normal for children to be slightly long sighted, this correction may assist those who have a marked tendency for long sightedness.

Malfunctioning STNR symptoms may include:

- A child crawling later than normal
- Poor hand-eye co-ordination
- An ape-like walking pattern
- Tendency to slump at a desk and/or poor posture due to a decrease in muscle tone, especially of the spinal muscles
- The eyes fatigue sooner than normal when focusing on near then far objects (copying from the blackboard may be slow and tedious, thus missing a lot of information gathered in class)
- Poor organisation and planning skills

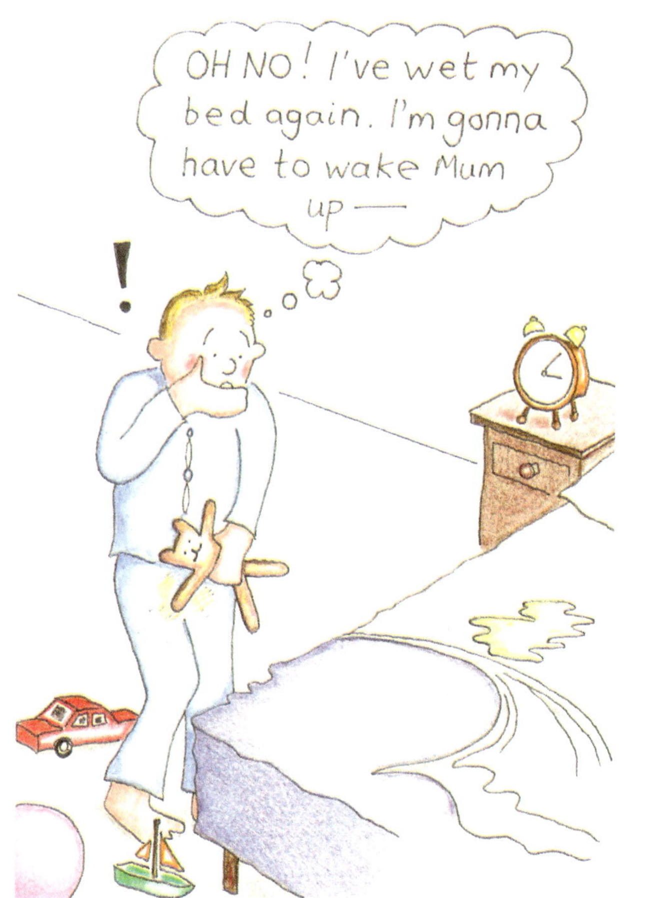

OH NO! I've wet my bed again. I'm gonna have to wake Mum up —

Suprapubic Reflex

The Suprapubic Reflex is present at birth. The reflex is elicited when pressure is detected at the pubic bones and the body responds by tipping the pelvis forward, straightening both legs. If the skin over one pubis is firmly touched, one hip moves backward and the other moves forward. The opposite pattern is seen in the upper body, enabling the baby to initiate commando crawling before the Symmetrical Tonic Neck Reflex activates to allow them to straighten their arms and legs to crawl on all fours.

There appears to be a firm association between a retained Suprapubic Reflex correction and bladder and kidney function, tone of the pelvic floor, and the reproductive system.

It seems also to link into one of the most ancient parts of the brain, the hypothalamus, which controls body temperature, appetite and sexual urges, and controls the glandular activity in the body, which regulates your unique biochemistry.

Suprapubic Reflex retention may lead to:

o   Bladder problems
o   Pelvic floor problems
o   Sugar handling imbalances
o   Imbalances in the hormonal systems
o   May affect walking pattern and posture
o   Difficult or recurring ankle, hip or shoulder problems

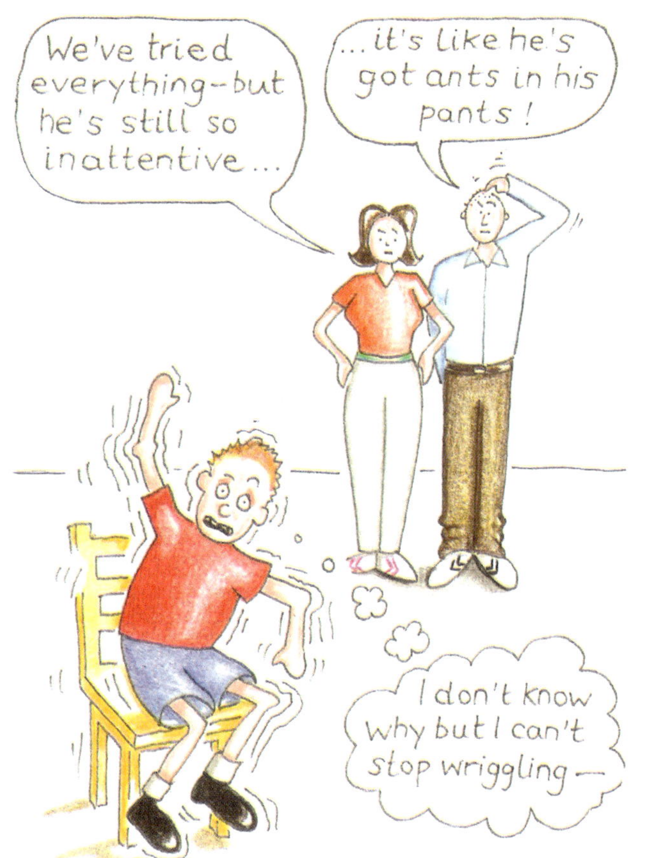

We've tried everything – but he's still so inattentive...
...it's like he's got ants in his pants!
I don't know why but I can't stop wriggling –

Spinal Galant

In a newborn baby, stroking the lower back on one side of the spine will result in side flexion of the lower back, with raising of the pelvis on that same side. It appears to take an active role in the birth process, with movements of the hip helping the baby to work its way down the birth canal.

Stimulation down both sides of the spine simultaneously will activate a related reflex, which causes urination.

If the Spinal Galant is retained it may be elicited at any time by light pressure on the lower back region, causing uncontrollable spinal movement.

The stimulation by bed sheets or pyjamas may activate the related urination reflex, causing bedwetting long after toilet training.

Spinal Galant retention may lead to:

- Inability to sit still (the 'ants in the pants' child who wriggles, squirms and constantly changes body position)
- Attention and concentration problems
- Difficulty co-ordinating normal walking movement
- Bladder control (bedwetting is common)
- Can contribute to the development of scoliosis (curvature) of the spine
- Clumsiness while trying to manipulate objects
- May affect fluency and mobility in physical activities or sports

Tonic Labyrinthine Reflex
Lack of concentration, difficulty sitting upright and motion sickness

Symmetrical Tonic Neck Reflex
Walking on toes, poor posture and co-ordination

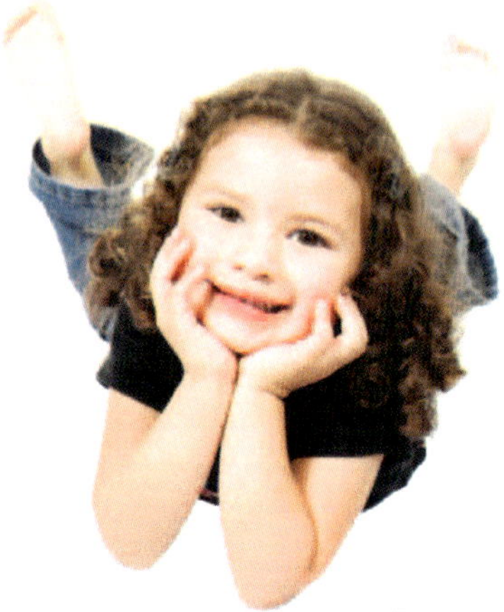

Fear Paralysis Reflex
Withdrawn, shyness, tantrums, anxiety

Moro Reflex
Over-reactive and over-sensitive (common in ADHD)

Asymmetrical Tonic Neck Reflex
Easily distracted, poor co-ordination and messy handwriting

Juvenile Suck and Rooting Reflexes
Speech, articulation and dental problems

Spinal Galant Reflex
Trouble sitting still and poor bladder control

Palmar Reflex
Jumbling up letters, poor writing expression and spelling, slouching at the desk/computer

Allied Therapies

The human body has an astonishing ability to heal. Miracles do happen and prior diagnoses can become obsolete. Children on the ASD spectrum can slide to the high functioning end, and children who were diagnosed as dyspraxic can end up winning more running races than anyone else in their school. Be ready to take the child out of the box he or she has been placed in.

The improvement in a child after RNR procedures alone can exceed expectations. In many cases they will bring about remarkable change without any other intervention, but these procedures were never intended to work alone. We encourage you to develop your network of allied therapists who work in other areas to assist in the development of growing bodies. For many patients further therapy is essential to relearn the skills to equip them for life.

Developmental delay and learning difficulty are multifactorial problems and therefore require a multidisciplinary approach to treatment. For decades RNR practitioners have worked alongside Behavioural Optometrists, Sound Therapists, Neurodevelopmental Assessors, Occupational Therapists, Medical Practitioners, Exercise Physiologists and Physiotherapists.

Your RNR practitioner can guide you to other practitioners whose approaches to assessment and care may be beneficial to your child. Many of the therapies have an association website which will give more information and may guide you to local practitioners.

The human body is masterfully capable of responding in a multitude of ways to incoming messages from the outer environment and its inner environment. The brain should fully collect and process incoming data and respond to the constant flow of messages with total ease, rectifying any glitches along the way. While an enhancement of even 10% in the body's ability to achieve this process may not be apparent immediately, observing the progressive accomplishments will allow parents to simply stand aside and applaud their successes. Let's allow your children to reach for the stars.

Notes